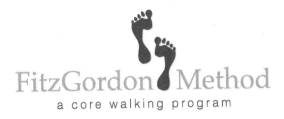

FitzGordon Method
a core walking program

The Spine: An Introduction To The Central Channel

D0595143

Jonathan FitzGordon

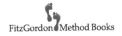

FitzGordon Method Books

Other books in this series:
Psoas Release Party!
Sciatica/Piriformis Syndrome
The Exercises of the FitzGordon Method

Although every effort has been made to provide an accurate description of posture remedies and their benefits, the information contained herein is not intended to be a substitute for professional medical advice, diagnosis or treatment in any manner.

Always consult your physician or health care professional before performing any new exercise or exercise technique, particularly if you are pregnant, nursing, elderly, or if you have any chronic or recurring conditions.

The authors are not responsible or liable for any injuries occurred by performing any of the exercises given or diagnosis made by a user based on the information shown within this document.

Cover Illustation: Frank Morris

TABLE OF CONTENTS

Copyright © 2011 Yoga Center of Brooklyn, LLC

I. INTRODUCTION:
AS THE SPINE GOES, YOU GO

"As the spine goes, you go." Bonnie Bainbridge Cohen, the creator of Body-Mind Centering.

Simple and true. The quality of your spine determines everything that works from it and around it. The solidity or the tone of your spine determines if your extremities work well, if your head works well, if your eyes work well, if your bowels work well. The spine is obviously central to our being.

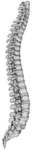

Illustation: Frank Morris

As humans, we have always known this. The spine is a central focus physically and symbolically across time and culture. In yoga there are three major energy channels – the sushumna nadi that runs up the spine and the ida nadi and the pingala nadi, which criss-cross around the spine. The idea of purification in yoga is about moving energy up from the base of the spine to the crown of the head through this sushumna nadi. The ida and pingala are

symbolized as snakes that wake up and move this energy. In doing so, they open each chakra. As you successfully purify or open the chakra, these snakes cross each other and move to the next one. Eventually this energy opens the thousand-petaled lotus, which explodes out of the top of the head.
Ah ha! Awakening!

Interestingly and probably not coincidentally, our Western medical caduceus uses similar imagery. There's a sword with snakes running up it. You see the main energy channel of the sword, the sushumna nadi, the spine. Then we have snakes wrapping around it like the ida and pingala, the nervous system. That sword and those snakes hold the integrity and energy of our spine, and thus the key to our integrity and energy as human beings.

In my work at the FitzGordon Method Core Walking Program, I tell people that the solidity and tone of the spine determines our health and well-being across body, mind and spirit. Again, "as the spine goes, you go."

In this book we'll look at the anatomy of the spine, some common spinal/postural issues and how to help them. More specifically we'll talk about the spinal curves and vertebrae, what happened when we went from four legs to two legs, the relationship between the spine and the pelvis as well as the spine and the extremities, how you don't need to shrink, how the spine affects the nervous system and movement and breathing, and of course our favorite topic – posture! With this information and accompanying exercises we aim to help you improve the quality of your spine and thus your life!

II. BREAKING DOWN THE SPINE

Your spine is made up of 24 vertebrae (ver-ta-bruh) that surround, protect and support the spinal cord. Each vertebrae can be seen as two halves, front and back—the body of the vertebrae facing front and the pedicles, lamina, and three jutting processes which form a ring making up the back half of the vertebrae. This ring creates the hole that the spinal cord passes through. The laminae are connected to the body of the vertebrae stalk-like structures called pedicles. The pedicles come off of the body of the vertebrae to connect with the lamina and processes. Using the diagram below, you can look at the spinal column as two distinct sections— the bodies of each vertebrae which stack to support and transfer weight, and then the processes coming off of the vertebrae body which allow for articulation, movement and connection to muscles. In the middle is the hole through which the spinal cord runs

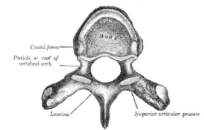

Illustration: Gray's Anatomy

In this diagram, you can see that there are two transverse processes on either side of the vertebrae where the back muscles connect to the spine. There is also a spinous process at the back, which is the bone you can see or feel down the center of someone's back. Often people think of this spinous process as the "spine" because that's what we see or feel. But each vertebrae has much more going on – these transverse processes that attach to the muscles that move you, and the body that supports and transfers weight.

So the spine is meant to support your weight. This is an important point because many of us have lost that flexibility and support of the spine. One of the main ways in which the spine supports us is with its brilliant spinal curves. The spine has four curves – two in and two out. Let's start from the bottom and move up, just like the upward movement of awakening energy in the yogic system.

We all have a tailbone leftover from when we had tails. This tailbone, the coccyx, looks like a little tail. It curves under a bit. This is the bottom tip of your spine. Some people can feel or sense the coccyx moving. For most of us, we only feel it when we land hard on our bums. If you've ever tried snowboarding chances are you met your coccyx! The silver lining to taking a fall like this is that you can now feel where the coccyx lives, deep in the body.

At birth the tailbone is made up of anywhere

from three to five bones that will fuse into one bone in the same way as the sacrum, which we'll get to next. But it's interesting to note that there remains an articulation between the sacrum and the tailbone. In fact, you can actually move your tailbone. One thing we'll discuss in this book is the importance of pelvic floor exercises to help us age gracefully, maintaining continence and a strong, balanced core. This articulation of the tailbone can be felt in such exercises. When you tone your pelvic floor you should feel that the tailbone moves closer to the pubic bone. The spatial relationship between the tailbone and the pubic bone is a key determinant of your core tone and thus your ability to remain continent (which we all care about) and strong as you age.

One of the many strange facts of life is we are drying up from the minute we are born. At birth we are about 80% water and by the time we die we are down to about 40% give or take. This natural desiccation has an extreme effect on our bones. Many of our joints ossify and fuse over time. The joint between the sacrum and the coccyx will fuse somewhere between the ages of 70 and 75. So whatever tone you have in the muscles of the pelvic floor when these bones fuse is the tone you will have the rest of your life! All to say that though it is small in size, the tailbone plays a large part in our health.

Up from the tailbone comes the sacrum, the first of the spinal curves. The sacrum curves out towards the back body. It consists of five vertebrae (bones of the spine). These are referred to as S1 through S5, with S5 being the bottom of the sacrum and S1 being the top. These sacral vertebrae begin as unfused (like the rest of the spine) when we are born. Once we being walking, the sacral vertebrae begin to fuse together to become more of a plate.

The sacrum is connected to the pelvis through two sacroiliac (SI) joints. These SI joints connect your spine to your pelvis and the legs. The sacrum moves within the SI joints with a minimal gliding motion. As a yoga teacher, I can get very insistent about the attempt to lengthen the sacrum down to move the tailbone in, but I often remind students that no matter how much I urge movement, it is an infinitesimal amount, 1/16 of inch at the most.

While the SI joints are not designed for much motion, that minimal amount of motion is key to healthy movement and ageing. All joints in the body are reciprocal and if one joint doesn't move with the others, the required movement is going to have to come from somewhere else. For example on a larger scale—the lower spine, the hip and the knee joint are all involved with walking but if your hip joint is "locked" or tight, the movement required of it will take place at either the knee or the lower back which is one of the reasons why we have so many injuries in those two areas (many of us are tight in the hips). You also need to have a balanced pelvis to allow for movement. Any deviation in the hips can easily lock the SI joint.

The SI joints are one of the many shock absorbers built into the body, absorbing shock from the spine and transferring weight to the pelvis and legs. In fact, this necessary movement in the SI plays a pivotal role in walking. The hip and sacrum solidify on each side with each step. They lock into one another to form a solid whole for each movement of the leg. Unless you study anatomy or movement you might never think of the sacroiliac joint or the sacrum but they are essential to our ability to move with ease.

Next up is the lumbar spine. This is a more commonly known area of the spine because many people experience back pain here. The lumbar spine curves in towards the front of the body. At least, it is supposed to curve in. However, too much curve, or a lack of curve, in this part of the spine is the cause of much of this back pain. The lumbar spine includes five vertebrae, L1 – L5. The lumbar vertebrae are the biggest and strongest of the spine. This makes sense intuitively. You can feel that this is your center of gravity. This part of the spine has the most access to flexion and extension. However, there is very little room for twisting because this action would compromise the lumbar spine's important role of bearing weight.

L5 is the bottom of the lumbar spine sitting right on top of S1. If you've read our Sciatica and Piriformis book, you know that the nerves that enervate your legs come together out of L4, L5, S1, S2, and S3. Knowing information like this helps you to get a sense of how connected everything is within your body. That pain in your knee or foot may be connected to a misalignment of your lower spine. What's wonderful about studying the spine is that its centrality helps you to understand the root of issues in the extremities, nervous system, balance, etc.

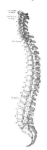

Illustration: Gray's Anatomy

Rising up from the lumbar spine, we come to the thoracic spine which naturally curves out towards the back body. The rib cage attaches to this part of the spine, forming a protective cage for the heart and lungs. Thus its alignment and tone are central to your breathing. Again, this basic anatomy can help you understand how your spine affects every aspect of your being. The thoracic spine has twelve vertebrae. T12 is right above L1, the top of the lumbar spine. T1 is all the way up where your neck begins.

The juncture of T12/L1 is a troubling one and the place where I see the greatest postural collapse in my clients. There is a big shift from the lumbar spine to the thoracic spine. First, the discs change shape, getting smaller as they go up. Plus, there is even a slight twist from L1 to T12. Finding the proper alignment of this area, known as the thoraco-lumbar joint, is a major step on the way to spinal health and is unfortunately very difficult to achieve.

An interesting thing to note here is the nature and alignment of the spinous processes. Function specifically follows form as the spinous processes determine just how much the spine can bend backwards. If you note the picture above, there is space between all of the spinous processes in the neck and lower back. They stick out and there is some room between them. When we look at the spinous process of the thoracic spine, they all lay directly on top of one another. This speaks to the rib cage protecting the heart and lungs, limiting the spines movement in this area.

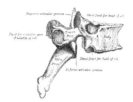

This is an important thing to note in yoga because I think a lot of people believe that when we backbend, much of it is coming from the upper back and chest when in fact there is no real bend in the thoracic spine. There is room for extension (lengthening) but no backward bending.

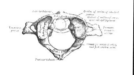 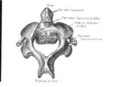 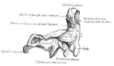

Atlas from above C1   Axis from above C2   Axis side view C2
Illustrations: Gray's Anatomy

This brings us to the final curve of the spine, the cervical curve. You can probably feel C7, the big vertebrae that sticks out and marks the base of the neck. C1 and C2 have a special shape and function and are responsible for much of the movement of the neck. Unlike all the other vertebrae, C1 and C2 don't have an intravertebral cushion between them. C2 is called the axis and it has a miniature pole, called the odontoid process, onto which C1, the atlas, sits. So the head sits on the atlas (C1), which sits on the axis (C2). The head and the atlas rotate around the axis. Thus this joint controls a great deal of the heads ability to move from side to side. Along with the SI joint and the thoraco-lumbar join, the atlas and axis make up the key spinal joints that are particularly vulnerable to disorder and dysfunction.

As such, the neck and throat are an area of tremendous importance to the body and your being. It is from the neck that we move our head and look out into the world. It is from the throat that we speak and connect with others. The health and stability of this part of the spine if vital to your connection and expression.

This cervical spine curves in toward the front body just like the lumbar spine. In fact, the cervical curve and lumbar curve are mirrors of each other. This means that the lower back and the neck are shaped in the same ways. They are designed to have the exact same degree of curve. As we will discuss in great detail, at the walking program we see a lot of people who tuck their pelvises under (removing the curve in the lumbar spine), which pushes the head forward (removing the curve in the cervical spine). You can imagine how the head forward and pelvic tucking habits have developed together in our culture. Moving our heads towards our computers or TV's, sinking into chairs and couches. A lot of our seemingly normal body positions are very unnatural to our magnificent bodies.

Knowing this basic anatomy of the spine and its curves can start you thinking about how you sit, stand and move and this is exactly the kind of awareness you need to live a vibrant, healthy life.

III. THE SPINE LENGTHENS
IN TWO DIRECTIONS

Now that we have the basics of the four spinal curves down, let's continue the anatomy discussion by looking at how the spine moves. There is a great deal of movement available to the spine, though each section moves differently. The spine can flex toward the front of the body, it can extend towards the back of the body; it can stretch to either side and can pull back to the middle from that side. It can rotate or twist as well though rotation is fairly limited in the lumbar spine while the cervical spine has a great deal of rotation. And as we said earlier there is not a lot of a backward bend available to the thoracic spine.

But let's take a look at how the spine lengthens energetically. This is way more interesting than the simple "stand up straight" from childhood.

First, it's worth looking at why we want to lengthen the spine. Sure, it could make you taller. But there's much more going on here. Again, energetically life revolves around the spine. The Central Nervous System (CNS) includes the brain and spinal cord, which is housed inside the spinal column. The Peripheral Nervous System (PNS) connects the CNS to other parts of the body, and is composed of nerves that emanate from the spinal column. Therefore, the skeletal alignment of our spine is the key determinant of our access to the body's energetic resources. Our nervous system is the body's information gatherer, storage center and control system. Its function is to collect information about external conditions in relation to the body's internal state, to analyze this information, and to initiate the proper response. It is our energetic mothership.

To unlock this energy we must balance the curves of the spine and lengthen them in two directions; the sacrum and tailbone move down, and the lumbar spine and everything above lifts up. We want to learn to lengthen the spine, while maintaining all of its natural curves in order to pull the spinal column to its maximum length. And, this is different than the throwing the shoulders back posture instruction that we are used to.

In order to visualize a healthy lengthening of the spine we need to understand the muscles that are involved in this action. Your pelvic floor is a group of muscles called the levator ani, (the elevator of the anus). Energetically these muscles move upward into the core of the body. Makes sense with the name. Your buttocks muscle, the big gluteus maximus, is a muscle that extends down the leg energetically flowing downward to the earth.

These muscles (levator ani & gluteus maximus) have specific functions that work in opposition to each other. Levator ani up. Gluteus maximus down. Unfortunately this is rarely the environment in which we live because we tend to overuse the buttocks and under use the pelvic floor and as a result the spine can begin to suffer. And as the spine suffers, we suffer. We create a compressed environment for the mothership of our nervous system.

In our experience at the walking program, we see that most people tend to overuse the buttocks. We grip in the buttocks when we're standing. Simply (and profanely put), we are a bit tight assed. How? If your legs are underneath your pelvis the butt can do less. However, we tend not to stand that way. Instead, we tuck the pelvis under while standing, just like when we're slouching in chairs. When the thighs begin to sink forward (as they do in most people), the quadriceps (big thigh muscles) and the buttocks must work to provide stability.

Gripping the buttocks shuts down energetic movement through the spine. In standing the gluteus maximus should not be working. Repeat. When you are standing, you should not be using your buttocks. Unfortunately, our buttocks-gripping posture usually shifts the gluteus maximus into a different role of sucking energy upwards rather than down. This means that our pelvic floor weakens because it's not able to do its real job of moving energy up.

An unfortunate result of these actions is that people are working their spine from the lumbar curve up instead of from the tailbone up. I see this in yoga class all the time. You can experience this in Cat & Cow (one of the exercises at the end). If you come onto your hands and knees and begin to arch and round the spine, you can try to feel where in the spine you initiate the action. We want to move from the tail all the way to the crown but I see that most people move from the lumbar up leaving the poor sacrum and tailbone out of the action.

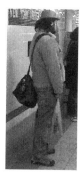

Releasing the buttocks opens the possibility for one of the body's most important features: toning the pelvic floor. Toning your pelvic floor creates the upward energy that allows for the sacrum and the tailbone to move down. Now toning your pelvic floor sounds way more interesting than throwing your shoulders back right? Yet, if the idea of toning your pelvic floor doesn't make sense you can try to feel it in many ways. Holding in your pee, gently engaging between the anus and the genitals and squeezing the anus to get a sense of movement at the base of the pelvis are but a few of many ways to feel your pelvic floor. Be patient and you will get it. Ideally you will feel a shift in the bones as well as the muscles. As mentioned earlier, when you tone your pelvic floor, your tailbone should move forward ever so slightly towards the pubis or front of the pelvis as the sacrum lengthens down. Add to this a gentle tone of the abdominals and a lengthening from the back of the neck can pull the spine up into its full extension at the top.

The key aspect of this is that though the spine is moving in two directions to find its length, the muscular action is all about lifting or lengthening up. It's about lifting the pelvic floor to release the lower spine down. In the chakra system, the tailbone is referred to as the root chakra. This is where our sense of stability and connection with the world originates. When we don't stand on our bones and we thrust the pelvis forward and grip the buttocks losing the tone of the pelvic floor—we lose our connection with the root or the earth. Sure, we might be able to lift up at bit through the upper spine, but everything below the lumbar spine is diminished. In that chakra system, the energy of the body originates at the base of the tail. We can't really lift up until we have this support. Thus, we need this harmonious relationship between the buttocks releasing down and the pelvic floor lifting up. Only then can the spine lengthen in two directions and create a healthy channel for our Central and Peripheral Nervous Systems. Only by moving in two directions can we create the space to energetically thrive.

IV. FROM FOUR TO TWO

But how did we even get to this miraculous place of a vertical spine? By exploring changes that occurred as we shifted from four legs to two legs, we can understand the mechanics of our modern body. So let's take a step back and look at what went down as we stood up.

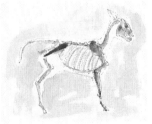

Illustration: Mark Chamberlain

Some serious changes had to occur for humans to step up to bi-pedalism. Look at a dog and you're looking at this horizontal spine that just sits into the bones of the pelvis. They don't even have a shoulder girdle. A horse's spine sits in this big web of fascia, and the spine can just hang down. Life is pretty easy for a spine that hangs down like that. It's not very hard to support the spine, and everything about gravity is working with the structure of the body.

Now the question of why we moved to two legs is the subject of endless evolutionary theories. I really like the theory that we had gotten to be tree dwellers and our brain start to grow bigger and larger. With that growth of the brain we needed a more complex diet than the trees were giving us. To get a more complex diet, we needed to cover more ground but we couldn't really do that on four legs. So evolutionarily we started to walk on two legs to get more complex foods to sustain the brain.

Also, if we went to the ground but stayed on four legs we'd be weaker than many four-legged predators. Perhaps two legs gave us an advantage and turned us from prey to predator. This theory is explored in the popular book Born To Run. Essentially we became running pack hunters. If we came down from the trees on four-legs, then we'd be taken out by four-legged predators who were tougher than we were. However, if we stood up then we could run. We could run for great distances as a pack, chasing a herd of antelope for example to wear down the most tired one. Then we could surround the animal, kill it, and get these complex nutrients for our growing brains. Watch a video of a pack of wolves working together to take down an elk and you'll get the picture. Now we aren't as fast as wolves. In Born To Run, the author argues that we had to be able to run great distances to wear down our prey. This means we were born to more than run; we were born to run ultramarathons. Food for thought.

So we came to two legs by necessity to successfully hunt and feed our brains. But on the way to standing up, all these major things happened. Let's start with the psoas. You may know that the psoas is my favorite muscle. Our first book is dedicated to the psoas. One of the reasons it is so important in human beings is that it's a major piece of the evolutionary bi-pedal puzzle. The four-legged creature doesn't have a working psoas. By this I mean that the psoas has nothing to do with their stability; it is a tender muscle for them. Literally, it is the tenderloin of a cow, the filet mignon. It doesn't touch the pelvis. But as we stood up, the psoas stretched across the pelvis. It became one of two muscles that attach our legs to our torso (piriformis is the other) and created our ability to be upright and stable. We'll have an entire chapter on the psoas and the spine in a bit. For now, we're just setting the scene on how essential this muscle is to our evolution and standing.

Also the gluteus maximus became a major player. The four-legged creature has no buttock. If you look at a cow you'll see what we call the sit bones (ischial tuberosities) sticking out and the leg flows down from there. They have no butt…the power of the gluteus maximus developed as it pulled down on the back of the pelvis, allowing the front of the pelvis to lift up taking the spine with it.

Releasing the buttocks opens the possibility for one of the body's most important features: toning the pelvic floor. Toning your pelvic floor creates the upward energy that allows for the sacrum and the tailbone to move down. Now toning your pelvic floor sounds way more interesting than throwing your shoulders back right? Yet, if the idea of toning your pelvic floor doesn't make sense you can try to feel it in many ways. Holding in your pee, gently engaging between the anus and the genitals and squeezing the anus to get a sense of movement at the base of the pelvis are but a few of many ways to feel your pelvic floor. Be patient and you will get it. Ideally you will feel a shift in the bones as well as the muscles. As mentioned earlier, when you tone your pelvic floor, your tailbone should move forward ever so slightly towards the pubis or front of the pelvis as the sacrum lengthens down. Add to this a gentle tone of the abdominals and a lengthening from the back of the neck can pull the spine up into its full extension at the top.

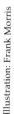

Illustration: Frank Morris

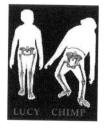

LUCY   CHIMP

The key aspect of this is that though the spine is moving in two directions to find its length, the muscular action is all about lifting or lengthening up. It's about lifting the pelvic floor to release the lower spine down. In the chakra system, the tailbone is referred to as the root chakra. This is where our sense of stability and connection with the world originates. When we don't stand on our bones and we thrust the pelvis forward and grip the buttocks losing the tone of the pelvic floor—we lose our connection with the root or the earth. Sure, we might be able to lift up at bit through the upper spine, but everything below the lumbar spine is diminished. In that chakra system, the energy of the body originates at the base of the tail. We can't really lift up until we have this support. Thus, we need this harmonious relationship between the buttocks releasing down and the pelvic floor lifting up. Only then can the spine lengthen in two directions and create a healthy channel for our Central and Peripheral Nervous Systems. Only by moving in two directions can we create the space to energetically thrive. This is one of our big evolutionary changes. Perhaps you've heard of Lucy, the famous skeleton of an early homo sapien. You see that the leg bones have started to change. They don't go out to the side. They are starting to go down. To be this upright we needed to develop an incredible solid pelvis. As we became more upright, the legs started going down from the pelvis rather than out to the side. They actually go down and in toward the knees. So now we have this big structure on top of these two little legs, which is a complete shift. No other creature has this set up.

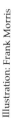

Illustration: Frank Morris

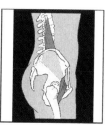

There is some genius architecture at work to let us do this, and it's about the gluteus maximus and the psoas, and the piriformis as we've said. That big, fat buttock muscle is the muscle that pulls us up to stand. Certainly the hamstrings (back of the leg muscles) help, but that big butt is what stood us up. It pulls us up and the spine comes upright. And in that standing, the psoas crosses the pelvis and is pulled into tension. When the psoas is pulled into tension, it then pulls the lumbar vertebrae forward because the psoas attaches to these vertebrae on the front and the side of the spine. This is how our lumbar curve is created. The downward pull of the glutes lifts the spine up…the psoas is stretched across the pelvis…in stretching it pulls the lumbar vertebrae forward and the piriformis provides a counterbalance at the back of the body connecting the outer leg to the sacrum. Now we can balance this big body atop our legs.

 www.FitzGordonMethod.com

Genius! That is the evolutionary creation of the lumbar curve…and thus the lumbar curve is everything! The curve of the lumbar spine determines its load bearing capacity. A well aligned spine has a lumbar curve that happily bears the weight of the rest of the spine, rib cage and head and successfully transfers that weight down through the sacrum into the pelvis all the way down to the feet. It is what helps us to stand and move as we uniquely do.

Unfortunately most people are using the lumbar curve terribly. Don't beat yourself up for that. We have bad posture because we can. We've been given this incredible lumbar curve. However, now instead of being slightly forward like apes, we're falling backwards into the lumbar curve. I think we are genuinely just confused about what it is to be upright with this new curve that nothing else ever had before.

V. TUCKING AWAY OUR EVOLUTION

Now that we understand a bit about our anatomy and how our posture came to be, let's explore our modern posture and how we're not working with the spine.

So when we stood up as a species, the psoas was awakened. This happens when we're children. When you learn to stand, the butt pulls down and hamstrings pull down and your spine is pulled up on top of your legs. Your psoas engages for the first time ever and this engagement pulls your lumbar spine into a natural curve.

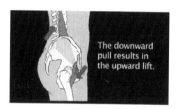

The downward pull results in the upward lift.

Illustration: Frank Morris

Now here is where things get really powerful. Your body is incredibly smart and employs reciprocal inhibition. This concept essentially means that muscles work in pairs, reacting to each other. For one muscle to lengthen its opposite must shorten and vice versa. When the psoas engages and pulls the lumbar spine forward into a natural curve, it is a downward motion. The psoas pulls down on the front of the lumbar spine. In order for you not to fall forward again, your genius body has an upward action happen on the other side of the spine. Your erector spinae muscles (which run vertically throughout the lumbar, thoracic and cervical regions) pull up. The psoas pulls down and the erector spinae muscles pull up. The cool thing here is that it is not likely that one muscle in and of itself can lift and support the spine and trunk. The psoas has to provide lift for the spine, through reciprocal inhibition, like we said but it needs help. The hipbone acts as a pulley and the psoas is the rope, thereby generating a much greater downward pull to allow for the heavy lifting the erector spinae muscle must employ for the spine to stay upright. With this strong frontward, downward pull of the psoas enough power is created for the erectors to extend up. Then your spine is set in beautiful tension to be held upright.

Now here's the modern posture tragedy! This power balance, this pulley of the psoas enabling the erectors to lift up is completely gone if you're tucking your pelvis. Just gone. Sadly this tucking is modern posture. It is an improper use of the psoas and it does not allow anyone's spine to live well. It gets worse though. Because now in all of modern exercise, modern athletics, modern movement, we are developing muscles around a spine and pelvis that is improperly aligned.

Illustration: Frank Morris

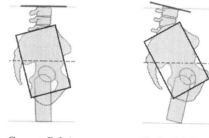

Correct Pelvis   Tucked Pelvis

Something happened and I'm not sure exactly when, but at a certain moment Doctors, Physical Therapists and their like started offering two contradictory solutions for lower back pain. One was to tuck the pelvis in order to create space in the lumbar spine and the other was to build your core muscles. The first instruction made an assumption that pain in the lower back was resulting from a problem with the pelvis rather than the trunk. My solution is the opposite- why not bring length to the lumbar from above rather than below. Not that it is easy but we think it is worth the effort.

Pain in the lower back most often comes from way we lean back into the lumbar curve, so that is what needs to be changed instead of positioning the pelvis incorrectly.

The second instruction for pain relief is often to strengthen the core. In and of itself this isn't a bad instruction but a number of things need to be taken into account. First and foremost, what is the position of the pelvis. If it isn't in the right place, as we mentioned earlier, you won't develop the core correctly. Another issue is which part of the core are you strengthening. Many people are told to do core work and start doing sit ups. Your sit ups muscle is called the rectus abdominus and is one of four abdominal muscles. As we'll go over later, if you aren't working all four of your abdominals equally you are doing a disservice to your trunk. Not to mention that your sit-ups muscle doesn't really have anything to with stabilizing your lower back. And if you have a tight psoas, building this muscle too much begins to squish the abdominal contents forward.

You might have powerful buttocks, you might have powerful abs, but if they're powerfully built to a pelvis that is tucked under, they're built all incorrectly. And that is why changing the posture is so difficult and that is why getting the muscles of the lower back to respond to all of these needs is so difficult.

Illustration: Frank Morris

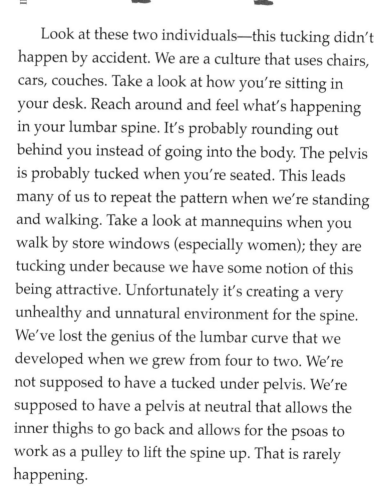

Look at these two individuals—this tucking didn't happen by accident. We are a culture that uses chairs, cars, couches. Take a look at how you're sitting in your desk. Reach around and feel what's happening in your lumbar spine. It's probably rounding out behind you instead of going into the body. The pelvis is probably tucked when you're seated. This leads many of us to repeat the pattern when we're standing and walking. Take a look at mannequins when you walk by store windows (especially women); they are tucking under because we have some notion of this being attractive. Unfortunately it's creating a very unhealthy and unnatural environment for the spine. We've lost the genius of the lumbar curve that we developed when we grew from four to two. We're not supposed to have a tucked under pelvis. We're supposed to have a pelvis at neutral that allows the inner thighs to go back and allows for the psoas to work as a pulley to lift the spine up. That is rarely happening.

This leads to an issue of imbalance. Balance is really the key to our posture as you can see already with the pulley system of the psoas and the erector spinae muscles. If the curve of the lumbar isn't there there's no way for the thoracic spine, the cervical spine and the head to sit successfully on top. Therefore your muscles are left searching for balance that they can't find.

We're in a chicken and egg situation with muscle alignment versus skeletal alignment. Because we have bad posture (skeletal alignment) our muscular alignment is awful, and we are imbalanced front to back. Our lower back muscles are incredibly short from this tucking under of the pelvis and habitually leaning backwards. Our hamstrings and quadriceps are completely thrown out of balance from this tucking under of the pelvis. Our erector spinae muscles are also short and tight because we are tucking under the pelvis and not using the psoas pulley system to lengthen them out and up. This imbalance also leads us to lose all core support and tone. Our muscles have developed this way because of our poor skeletal alignment (not using our lumbar curve). Now that our muscles are developed as such, if you put yourself into correct skeletal alignment in the pelvis, the muscles just pull you back into imbalance. It's an unfortunate trap.

What I've found with my yoga students and walking program clients is that reclaiming your body from this trap is a combination of releasing, stretching, strengthening and toning. People often think that if they have low back pain or poor posture there are sit-ups to do or a pulling back of the shoulders. But there's much more subtle and interesting work to do with the core and pelvis to bring back your natural, glorious spinal curves. We'll get to specific exercises at the end of this book. For now though let's hope the seed is planted that what you'll be doing is uncovering your body's genius. The evolution is there in our architecture. We simply need a postural revolution to start standing up again.

VI. EVERYTHING'S CONNECTED

As part of the posture revolution, let's look at how the spine works with our extremities. Here's the short version – our extremities aren't all that connected to the spine! The connections are fairly minor, so our body is actually relying on a very stable spine and trunk or core. All the more reason to get that posture correct.

Now this stable spine isn't about strength. It's about balance as we've been discussing – muscle balance, skeletal balance. We have beautiful architecture so that we don't have to rely on strength. Let's say we have a beautifully balanced trunk, a powerful trunk. There's really not a lot connecting the extremities to this trunk.

SPINE AND THE LEGS

Let's start with the legs. They are connected to your spine by only the psoas and the piriformis. That's it. Think about it. There are only two muscles connecting your legs to your spine...and many of us don't even know these muscles exist. These muscles are so important that they are the subjects of our first two books.

Illustration: Frank Morris

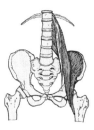

The psoas connects in the front of the spine as we've mentioned. This can be difficult to visualize. Imagine your spine running up through your body. You have the back side of it, which you can feel with your hand along your back. We don't often think about the front side of the spine behind the abdominal organs. But there it is and the psoas originates at the last thoracic vertebrae (T12) and the first four lumbar vertebrae (L1, L2, L3, L4). So we can see how the psoas would pull the lumbar forward into it's beautiful curve. The psoas crosses across the pelvis and attaches on the inside of your femur (the large thigh bone).

The psoas is the main flexor of the leg. Flexing is when we draw the leg closer to the chest. We do this action on a small scale each time we step the foot out in front of us. Many people think the quadriceps is doing or initiating the walking but it is really an extensor of the knee. You can feel this by putting your hand on your thigh and taking your knee up towards your hip. The quadriceps will be relaxed. Now straighten your leg and you will feel the quadriceps engage.

Therefore, the psoas is the main muscle for walking. It is also the main muscle for trauma. Anytime you are afraid, you flex. Imagine yourself as an animal in nature. If you played dead, the psoas would draw the knees in to the chest. If you wanted to fight, the psoas helps you get small and spring up. If you wanted to run, the psoas moves your feet forward. When the fear responses kicks in, the psoas goes into action.

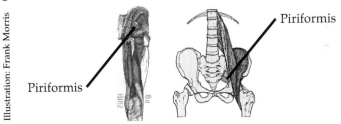

Illustration: Frank Morris

Piriformis

Piriformis

The other muscle attaching the leg to the spine is the piriformis. The psoas attaches the leg in the front and the piriformis in the back. The piriformis connects to the front or anterior portion of the sacrum, the lower part of the spine. Unlike the psoas, the piriformis doesn't cross in front of the pelvis. It travels from the sacrum passing through the sciatic notch and then attaches to the outside of the large thigh bone (the femur). So the psoas and the piriformis act like a stirrup of sorts attaching the leg to the spine in the front and the back of the body.

The piriformis is a tiny muscle. But it greatly affects the movements of your legs, hips, and spine.

The tone and balance of your piriformis (on each side) is tremendously important to the body and your movement. One reason we lose tone in the piriformis is this unfortunate tucking posture. A large majority of people stand and walk with their feet turned out (again, shortening the back body). Anatomical neutral, which would hopefully be our default posture, has the feet close to parallel. This stance of the feet creates the ideal resting position for the piriformis. You can feel this when standing. With the feet parallel the buttocks can be broad and untucked more easily. If the feet are turned out the piriformis is automatically shortened into a contracted state. If this is your natural posture and walking pattern your piriformis is slightly contracted 24/7, which compromises the position of the spine.

SPINE AND THE ARMS

When it comes to the arms, the connection situation is even more tenuous. The only muscle connecting the arms to the spine is the latissimus dorsi...known as the lats. The lats are a massive muscle that connect all the way down to your pelvis. So while just this one muscle connects, it is enormous (latissimus means broad). Anatomically there is an interesting twist to the lats- the insertion is literally twisted when the arm is down by your side. It untwists when the arm lifts which increases both its ability to stretch and generate force. It can pull the body up for climbing or depress the arm against resistance. Another way of looking at it is the lats are our swinging from the trees muscle.

Let's go back to evolution and the shoulder. When the first creatures slithered out of the primordial muck to move along the earth, arms developed and the full weight of the body sat on the shoulder and "arm". As creatures evolved and moved up into the trees to swing from branches our entire body was hanging from the arm. So we have moved from compression to suspension and finally freedom as now the arm hangs from the shoulder, free to move in any and every direction.

In our minds two main things are restricting this freedom— a tucked pelvis, and the age old instruction "take your shoulders back". This is the essence what is known as military posture as well as Mom's classic lament, and unfortunately from my perspective an essential instruction of most yoga teachers. All three of these disrespect the amazing freedom the shoulder allows us.

The arm is meant to hang from the shoulder. This is key to upright posture and especially key to optimal functioning. If your pelvis is tucked under the shoulder joint is restricted. Feel free to try it. Tilt the top of your pelvis forward a bit and see if you feel the hang of the arm. Tuck under and feel it disappear. The same restriction occurs when we jam the arms back to "stand up straight" for better posture. Good posture is determined by a free swinging arm. You can't have one without the other.

To mix it up a bit more, most people have an upside down view of the design of the body. It isn't unreasonable. You would think that the head sits down on top of the spine, the shoulder girdle on top of the rib cage, pelvis on top of the leg, etc, and to some degree this is obviously true.

But the body is really a series of hanging structures from the head down. Your shoulder girdle (collarbones and shoulder blades) connects to the rib cage in one spot, where the collarbone meets the rib cage. Other than that it should sit suspended over the ribs cage, hanging from muscles that connect it to the head.

The arm hangs from the shoulder as mentioned and the lower leg hangs from the pelvis in its way. We are a complicated machine.

All you have attaching the shoulder girdle to the spine is the rhomboids, which is just an amazing thing. The shoulder girdle only connects in one little spot skeletally at the front where the clavicle meets the sternum. So the rhomboids are the only thing connecting the shoulder girdle to the spine. This seems almost unbelievable, but it's all about muscle balance.

The rhomboids need some attention in this spine conversation because our modern posture patterns do some strange stuff up here. Generally speaking, I say we are tight in the back and loose in the front. Again, see the pelvis tucking under and how that shortens your lower back and collapses your core support. This pattern changes in the upper back. Most everyone is loose and weak in the rhomboids and short and tight in the front of the chest. When the lumbar collapses, the thoracic spine rounds backwards and the cranium goes forwards. That adds to the story of our bad posture.

What's interesting is that everyone thinks they're rounded in the upper chest. They are. However, they're rounded backwards in a weird way because the upper back moves backwards and the upper chest rounds forward. But they're not leaning forward in a way I think most people perceive they are. This position pulls the shoulder blades off the back and stretches the rhomboids with them. The shoulders are rounded off the back and this shortens the muscles at the front of the chest, the pectoralis major and minor (the pects). This important imbalance shows the rhomboids being loose and the pects being tight. In Rolfing words they call it locked long and locked short.

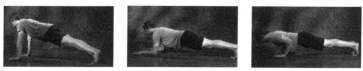

Perhaps you're familiar with the plank position, which is often used in yoga. It's a great place to illustrate this issue. One of the main things I'm trying to teach people in plank and in forearm plank is that if your upper back is round (pushed up) then you're only using your pectoral muscles (in the front of the body) to hold you up. You're not using your abs nearly as much as you can. These poses are a great opportunity to strengthen the abs and the core, but most of us miss it. I'm trying to teach people to soften the upper back.

Notice the groove between the shoulder blades in the pictures above, in an attempt to bring balance between the pects at the front of the chest and the rhomboids on the back. If you can soften the upper spine down to stop using the pects as much, you should then feel the abdominals kick in like crazy. But again, it's not about strength, it's always about balance, balance, balance.

In fact, let's talk about balance between these two muscles that are connecting our legs and arms to the spine. One of my heroes, Ida Rolf said, "The only thing that matters is the connection of the psoas and the rhomboids." Now she never really explained herself on that one. But here's where I think she was going with this – in a lot of ways the psoas is strapping your spine in at the front of the body with the legs and the rhomboids are strapping your spine in on the back of the body with the shoulder girdle

If you're solid, balanced, and toned, then the extremities can move with ease. If your trunk isn't in the right place and your pelvis isn't in the right place, then things won't work well. So the quality of the spine, the quality of the center, the quality of the trunk determines everything the extremities can or can't do. More and more we see that the spine is the key to unlocking fluid, easy movement in the body. The exercises provided at the end of this book will help you to bring your body back to a place of natural ease for life.

VII. YOU DON'T HAVE TO SHRINK

Speaking of lifelong natural ease, did you know that we don't have to shrink as we get older? We all assume that we'll get a bit shorter as we age. But that doesn't have to be by much. We can remain gloriously upright if we work with nature.

Let's look at what is causing the shrinking. We've mentioned that the spine is made up of vertebrae, which are bones. We've discussed the sections of the spine – sacrum, lumbar, thoracic and cervical. Each of these sections is made up of vertebrae. The bones are stacked atop each other. Again, our natural curves help to balance us in this historically unprecedented upright position

In between these bones are fluid sacs called intervertebral discs. There are actually lots of fluid sacks throughout the body, not just between the vertebrae. It's one of the ways in which is body is so fluid filled. Perhaps you've heard the term bursa or bursitis? A bursa is a fluid sack that helps joints glide and we have bursas all over the body facilitating the movement of our joints. Bursitis is when a fluid sack becomes swollen or inflamed. All to say, these sacks are alive and changing and responding to how we move our bodies. The intervertebral discs provide a cushion for the spine between the boney vertebrae.

These discs are fluid filled, and they're like pillows.

It's a pretty simple image. Imagine that you have a level surface and then a water balloon on top. Then you set a heavy book on top of the water balloon. The balloon is going to squish a bit right? And if you pressed on one side of the book or one corner of the book, the balloon under that bit would decompress and the side opposite it would get larger. There's fluidity and movement and change.

There is also fluidity, movement and change within our spine. Our discs are like this water balloon. If you lean backwards, then the back side of your vertebrae will push on the back side of the disc, just as the book would with the water balloon. When this happens, then the front of the fluid-filled disc will squish out a bit. That is what we're doing to these very tender, fluid-filled sacks all the time.

Eventually that's what leads to a herniation. We have repetitive motions in our posture and movements, and after time and pressure that fluid sack can pop out and not squish back into even alignment. If this happens to you, it is not a final sentence for the spine and your core strength. There are ways to find relief whether through release work, bodywork and or stretching, help is out there. Of course this takes time, patience and consistent work.

However, herniation is a special case. We all experience change (and squishing!) in our discs over the course of the day. The biggest change is their decompressing. Think about what happens when you lay down in bed at night and put your head on the pillow. The pillow might feel really thick and you think it's too much. But within a few minutes it's mellowed out, and it's much more comfortable for your head.

The same exact thing is happening to your discs over the course of your day. When you go to sleep your discs relax, your spine relaxes, you lay down horizontally and everything says 'ahhhh' and you grow about a quarter of an inch. And then, after you get up the next morning, you basically spend the day shrinking that quarter of an inch because of the way you put pressure onto these discs.

That's what gravity is doing. It's banging down on us all the time. What's interesting about gravity is the quality of our health and the quality of our life is really about the way we work with gravity. If you're working with gravity, your joints are not going to suffer and, in large part, because your fluid sacks are not going suffer. Working with gravity simply means standing and moving with proper alignment. When you stand the way we're instructing (i.e., using the curve in your lumbar spine), then you are even. When you walk well, you walk with gravity. You're using your body's natural intelligence and you're working with gravity.

Here's another cool image around this notion of gravity. If you go to space (and thus aren't subjected to gravity), you will grow a couple of inches. When people return from space, they are sequestered so they can shrink back to Earth size! Besides the wow factor of that factoid, the amazing thing is that our spine has all this room for elongation. That's a healthy, wonderful thing. When I'm instructing walking or yoga, I will give alignment points to help people lengthen the spine. So when everyone says, "well you shrink two inches over the course of your life," that doesn't have to be the case. Sure, you'll shrink a bit each day over the course of the day but then you'll lengthen out again at night. You don't have to permanently shrink. You can even create more space if you improve your alignment and movement patterns. Perhaps you could get taller as you age!

A balanced musculature helps to minimize the compression that our body goes through each and every day. If the abdominal muscles all have their proper tone, they will maintain an appropriate space between the pelvis and the rib cage. This is one of their jobs.

Here's a really interesting tidbit – that lost height unfortunately means lost space for your organs and nerves. My mother just had a hip replacement. I took her to a neurologist to make sure her nerves were working pre-op. The doctor and she discussed how she was now 5'6" but used to be 5'8". He said, "Well your nerves don't shrink, only your height does." Thus one of the reasons many people begin to have nerve damage and impingements as they age is simply because there is less space. However, if you keep your muscle tone, preserve good alignment and work with gravity, you don't have to suffer when you hit 70 and 80.

It's all about tone and alignment, which is great because you can work to improve that. So you don't have to shrink. You can keep your height and preserve your space.

VIII. NERVES AND THE SPINE

While we're addressing the nervous system, let's look more specifically at an important relationship between the spine and the nerves. You have the central nervous system, the brain and the spinal cord, and you have the peripheral nervous system, which is everything that comes out of the spinal cord. If the spine is well aligned, and only if the spine is well aligned, will the peripheral nervous system work well. Simple as that.

The nervous system runs the show. Nothing happens without the nervous system's go ahead, and many physical ailments stem from its disorder and misalignment.

Every little impingement of a nerve affects its ability. Think about being outside with a garden hose. You control the flow of water by crimping the hose and can shut the flow off completely by bending it. This is very similar to what is going on with your nerves. If you crimp a nerve a little bit, you get issues like numbness in the feet, no circulation in the hands or feet. It's all about alignment. When the spine is well aligned, the nerves flow. You have space and length, the nerves flow. That is simple, basic, and clear.

The subtler and perhaps more surprising relationship between the spine and the nerves is really about the spine and the eyes. Here's the basic deal – your spine moves because your eyes tell it to move. Your eyes are relaying with the brain and telling the spine how to move. The vital connection for this movement is the sub occipital muscles, four small muscles connecting the head to the top of the spine.

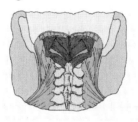

Illustration: Frank Morris

Wondering where those are? Try this little exercise. Close your eyes and dig your thumbs into the base of your skull. Keeping the eyes closed, move them peripherally. With your thumbs, you can feel your sub occipital muscles moving when your eyes move. They are the only muscles in your body connected to the eye…and the eye is the nervous system's only connection to the outside world. So these sub occipital muscles are incredibly important to your health and movement.

You know the story about how a cat lands on all fours no matter where you drop it from? It's doing that because of the eye's relationship to the sub occipital muscles. The inner ear registers balance and then the eye registers level. The eye tells the sub occipital "fire," and the sub occipitals initiate an extension of the spine so the cat can land on all fours. The same exact thing is happening in our spine with every step we take. Through the sub occipital muscles, the eyes are communicating to the spine how to move.

Illustration: Frank Morris

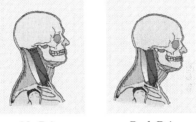

No Pain   Back Pain

We run into problems because most everyone is tight in the sub occipital muscles. We've discussed how tucking our pelvis throws our spine out of alignment and often leads to a forward head posture. The main muscular issue in forward head posture is the sub occipitals because they connect the atlas and the axis, the two vertebrae on top of the spine. They are shifted forward and the muscles connecting the spine to the eyes are off. You won't move through space well if your eyes and spine can't communicate. The efficacy of movement is diminished if the connection between the eye and the spine are thrown out of kilter. We'll offer exercises at the end on lengthening the sub occipitals. You need to learn how to lengthen those muscles; again you want to create space.

These cramped, tight sub occipital muscles hamper our walking. I often teach people to walk looking at the horizon line. It's an attempt to get their heads on straight, so to speak. You have to look straight ahead to make this connection between your eyes and your sub occipitals. But instead, everyone's chin is elevated and they're looking down. Their eyes are tilting down to look straight ahead because they think that's what straight ahead is.

Ancient marathoners would use the horizon line to run. The stride becomes easier because the eyes and spine are communicating well. Then they can get lost in the meditation of the motion; the body doesn't have to work as hard. The same goes for you and walking. You don't have to waste energy and can move efficiently instead. The nervous system will work better. Everything comes back to alignment. If you have good alignment, you don't have to work as hard and the body will operate better...for much longer!

More and more we can see that spinal alignment is about much more than good posture. It is vital to how you move through the world.

IX. BALANCE IS POWER

Good spinal alignment isn't simply about putting everything into place. You need muscle tone to keep it there. There's an interesting relationship between the spine and the trunk. Think about how there are so many bones in the body. And then there's a section between the pelvis and the rib cage where there aren't many bones. There are five bones between the pelvis and the rib cage. The only other support there is muscle, along with fascia, ligaments and tendons.

This means that it truly is the muscle tone between the pelvis and the rib cage that goes a long way in determining our posture and our movement patterns. In my experience with walking clients and yoga students, this is the tightest area of the body and one of the hardest places to work.

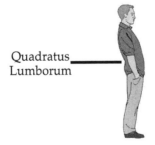

Quadratus Lumborum

Illustration: Frank Morris

The psoas was the focus of our first book so we won't delve too deeply into it here, but we will look at muscles of the trunk that surround it and are affected by it. First, is its next door neighbor the quadratus lumborum. This is a side bending muscle that connects the pelvis to the rib cage. It either draws the trunk down to the side or lifts the side of the pelvis up. These muscles are bedeviling to body workers and yoga teachers. They tend to be incredibly tight if you fall into the posture pattern of long in the front and short in the back. If you are leaning backwards with the shoulder behind your hips like the picture above (and I can almost guarantee that you are) these muscles are going to be habitually and chronically tight. They can and will open but from my experience they are some of the hardest muscles to lengthen and release.

Next we'll look at muscles deep in the spine. There are several layers of muscles deep inside the back (intertransverse, interspinalis, transversospinalis, semispinalis, mulitifidus & rotatores) running up and down the spine connecting in all manner of crosshatched patterns. They connect from tranverse process to transverse process, from spinous process to spinous process as well as from the transverse process to the spinous process. They all aid and assist in flexing, bending and rotating.

The next, or middle, layer of back muscles are called the erector spinea (iliocostalis, longissimus, spinalis). These muscles along with the transversospinalis lengthen or extend the spine up in connection with the engagement of the psoas that pulls the lumbar spine forward. As the psoas pulls the lumbars vertebrae forward these spinal muscles do the opposite, thereby lengthening to spine to its fullest.

Look back to the perils of bad posture. All of these deep spinal muscles work together and require tone in one to have tone in all. Consequently when the lower back muscles are short and tight these chains of spinal muscles will not be able to extend up because at their base they lack tone to assist their relatives higher up.

Many people are really, really tight. I've seen walking clients who will have to scream to stretch a muscle. They'll be trying to stretch the calves and shouting, "ahhhh!". To get out of that tightness requires more than just stretching. It requires core work and not only core strengthening. It gets a little complicated when we talk about this because people think "core" and think "strengthen". But it's actually about balance. Ida Rolf would say that people would come to her and talk about how strong they are; she would tell them that strength is meaningless and balance is everything. Balance is power.

The pattern we see most in our culture is tight in the back and weak in the front. I can't tell you the amount of clients who have come to me with back problems who say they went to doctors, physical therapists, etc. who say, "well you have back problems, you have to do core work." But that could make matters worse. They are tight in the back and their psoas is tight. So they are pushing their abdominal contents forward, they believe the doctor so they start doing a thousand sit-ups or crunches. This tightens the abdominals, which means all they're doing is really crunching all the contents of their abdomen and their intestines and stuff. This doesn't help anything and really hurts your abdominal organs and even your back. Space equals health. You need to go for balance.

The muscle balance that's key for the health of the spine (and for the psoas) is our holy trinity of muscle groups – pelvic floor, abdominals, and inner thighs. When we're talking about the spine, the importance of the pelvic floor cannot be overemphasized. It's connected literally to the base of the spine at the tailbone, the base of the pelvis at the sit bones (ischial tuberosities) and at the pubic bone (we'll share exercises for these muscles at the end).

Our pelvic floor is not only intimately connected with eliminative issues, it is also responsible for bearing the weight of the organs that sit above it. Lack of tone in these muscles, called the levator ani, prevents us from having a stable pelvis, and without a stable pelvis, we are not likely to have a happy spine.

If you are someone who has done a great deal of sit-ups and not as many pelvic floor lifts, you are likely looking at a pretty severe muscle imbalance. The pelvic floor, which connects from the tail bone to the pubic bone, essentially continues as the rectus abdominus (sit ups muscles), which runs from the pubic bone to the base of the rib cage.

The rectus abdominus is one of four abdominals. These muscles are separate and not separate. They connect through fascia (a webbing connecting all parts of the body) which forms the linae alba at the front and they connect through the thoraco-lumbar fascia at the back. They are bound together yet have separate roles. That reality demands balance if any of them are to work correctly.

But the transverse abdominus are the most important in terms of the spine. It's the only one that basically connects into the lumbar. Granted it connects into the fascia and the connective tissue at the lumbar, but it is the only of the abdominals that wraps from the back to the front in its engagement. For me this means that tone in the transverse abdominus is required for stabilizing the lumbar spine. So, while all of the four abdominals are really key to the support of the trunk, only one, transverse abdominis, is really connected to the stability of the lumbar spine. And proper tone in the transverse will help bring balance to all four abdominal muscles. This is the key muscular answer for relieving back pain. It isn't alone on the road to healing but it often leads the way.

This is where people get into trouble thinking that if you have back problems that you should do a lot of sit ups. Those are the work of the rectus abdominis, and that's the most superficial muscle. The rectus helps you do crunches and it's important to be balanced there, but it doesn't help with stabilizing the lumbar. In fact, an overly contracted, tight rectus would lengthen the lumbar and remove the important curve. The rectus shortens the distance between the pelvis and the rib cage in two directions. It both pulls the pelvis up and the rib cage down. An overly developed rectus pulls the pelvis into an unnatural tuck. It also lengthens the lumbar spine, which can be positive as space is good. But the rectus is not working to stabilize the lumbar spine. A lot of body workers like massage therapists and rolfers refer to the "tyranny of the rectus abdominis". The rectus takes over at the expense of weakening the other abdominals.

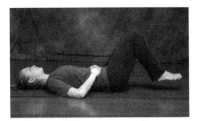

I see this a lot in my work as well. I'll ask people to access the transverse by simply taking one foot off of the floor and then the other with the knees bent (see the photo above). This is a very basic exercise. But they don't usually use the transverse; they access the rectus. This usually manifests in either the belly popping up on engagement or the lumbar spine lifting and arching too much. They keep accessing the rectus until finally they'll start getting to the transverse. This imbalance highlights the work many people need to do. How do you get out of a muscle that doesn't support the spine to a muscle that does. Of course we'll address this with the exercises at the end of the book. We'll help you to access the transverse, so you can create functional strength and support for the spine. We'll help to balance you in your trunk.

We'll also provide exercises for the two other abdominal muscles the internal and external obliques. While we don't consider these muscles intrinsic to the issues of most back pain, the lack of balance in the whole muscle group always has an effect.

Your trunk is your center. All of this talk of "core strength" in society is a good thing. We want to move from the center; we want to support the spine. But we want to do this in a smart way so that our body is truly intelligent.

X. BREATH IS LIFE

If balance is power, then breath is life. Proper alignment of the spine facilitates both. Yes, proper alignment of the spine keeps you alive. If your spine is in the right place, then you can get clear, efficient breath. Breathing should be easy. In fact, in our way of thinking living in your body should be easy.

We talked about how you want your head to be level. Similarly you want your diaphragm and pelvic floor level as well. You can think of these as three platforms in the body. They mirror each other just as the curve in the neck mirrors the curve in the lower back. With a proper curve in the lumbar spine and neck, these three platforms can be level.

In fact, the pelvic floor and the diaphragm are synergists. They do the same thing at the same time. When you inhale, the diaphragm drops to make space in the lungs and the pelvic floor drops as well. This dropping of the diaphragm moves the abominal organs forward and the belly pushes out a bit. Many of us do something called reverse breathing. The diaphragm gets stuck when we inhale, puffing the chest up and out. In doing so, we don't allow ourselves full, complete inhales. In the natural inhaling process, the belly pushes out a bit as the diaphragm drops down. Place your hands on your belly and spend a few moments trying to find natural breathing – belly out on the inhale. You can imagine your pelvic floor relaxing down as well. They work together.

This means that the belly comes in on the exhale as the diaphragm rises. The pelvic floor lifts as well. Try doing a kegel (gentle squeezing and lifting the pelvic floor muscles as if you were stopping your urine flow) during an exhalation. It's pretty natural. Now try to squeeze and lift that area when you inhale. It's tough. Because your pelvic floor is moving with the diaphragm when you inhale; they are both dropping down. And when you exhale, they both rise.

Of course you need proper muscle tone for the pelvic floor and diaphragm to move together. It gets back to the holy trinity of the pelvic floor, abdominals and inner thighs. The intelligent core strength. The muscles that need to work as synergists aren't going to do so of their own accord. They need help from toned muscles around them to keep them in the right place so that they can work as synergists.

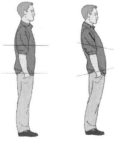

Illustration: Frank Morris

You also need proper spinal alignment. Because we've tucked our pelvis under, we tend to lean backwards a bit…as if to find the natural curve and balance that the lumbar would give us if we used it. We lean back right at the top of the lumbar spine where it meets the thoracic spine (L1 and T12 in vertebrae speak). This is a very important juncture point in the body – the psoas and the trapezius both connect there. This is the level of the diaphragm and the solar plexus. We're leaning backwards and compromising this important physical and energetic center. Of course this also makes us round the upper back backwards and the upper chest forward. (To be fair, before you collapse into self-judgment, remember the images our culture promotes…butts under, abs in, shoulders up and back). This postural issue is a big reason why we're reverse breathing, compromising our breath capacity and efficiency. When we inhale in this position, the diaphragm hits the spine. The diaphragm just drops right onto the shelf that you created by leaning backwards. It has nowhere else to go.

Play with this change. Allow yourself to have a curve in your lumbar and then drop your front ribs (the ones you can see sticking out, just give them a pat so they fold into the body). Breathe in this place. Do you feel how the belly pushes out a bit? The breath falls more naturally into the entirety of the lungs and the diaphragm moves down pressing the belly out a little. That change to the spinal alignment makes everything work better…including breathing and thus being alive.

XI. PROBLEMS OF THE SPINE

We have established the importance of the spine, and its need for proper alignment and tone. But before we move into solutions and exercises, let's touch briefly on some common spinal issues. It is my belief that the more information we have at our fingertips the more likely we are to heal. Too many people suffer through conditions without fully understanding what they are going through. Here is a short synopsis of some of the issues that many people are saddled with.

- **Psoas Pain** is related to the psoas manifests in myriad ways. Hip pain, groin pain, lower back pain, a wrapping pain from the pubic bone to the outer hip and lower back pain are all possible symptoms of psoas issues. The psoas is the subject of our first book so we will point you in that direction for more information and exercises.

- **Sciatica/Piriformis Syndrome** - Sciatic pain usually emanates from the lumbar spine and ends in a shooting pain down your leg. The piriformis muscle attaches to the base of the spine on the front portion of the sacrum and piriformis syndrome most always manifests as a pain in the deep buttocks that radiates down the leg. Our second book is on sciatica and piriformis syndrome and, again, we suggest you turn there for more discussion and exercises.

- **Spinal Disc Herniation**, often referred to as a "slipped disc", is a condition in which a fissure in the outer ring of an intervertebral disc lets the soft middle seep out. Imagine that water balloon again (your disc), but let's fill it with jelly. A fissure in the outer layer would allow that jelly to begin leaking out. Discs almost always slip to the side (leak out the side) due to strong ligaments lining the back of the spine. Most herniations in the lower back happen between the fourth and fifth lumbar vertebrae or between the fifth lumbar vertebrae and the sacrum. This is right where the sciatic nerve originates.

- **Degenerative Disc Disease** is not really a disease but a term used to describe changes in the spinal column as you age. Between each vertebra there is the above mentioned disc, a soft cushion that acts as a shock absorber for the spine, allowing it to flex, bend, and twist. Poor posture and bad movement patterns can lead to a degeneration or wearing down of the discs, which in turn can lead to a host of other problems.

- **Spinal Stenosis** is a narrowing of the spine occurring most often in the neck or lower back. This narrowing can put pressure on the spinal cord or spinal nerves at the level of compression. Spinal stenosis is commonly thought to be caused by age-related changes in the spine. As always we feel that poor mechanics and conditioned patterns have more to due with the body's breakdown that anything else. In severe cases of spinal stenosis, doctors perform surgery to create additional space for the spinal cord or nerves.

- **Spondylolysis and Spondylolisthesis** result from a weakness in a section of the vertebra called the pars interarticularis, the thin piece of bone that connects the upper and lower segments of the facet joints. Facet joints link together the upper and lower joints of the vertebrae to form a working unit that permits movement of the spine. The pars interarticularis is found in the posterior (back) of the vertebra. Spondylolysis occurs when there is a fracture of the pars portion of the vertebra. Spondylolisthesis occurs when the vertebra shifts forward due to instability from the pars defect. I believe that this type of injury is most commonly caused by conditioned patterns and habits. When the structural alignment of the spine is not working optimally, the environment for stress fractures increases exponentially.

- **Scoliosis** afflicts many people , even if just a touch. Many of them will never even know they have a bit of scoliosis. As beings of nature, we are asymmetrical. So it makes sense that our spine would be as well. However, much of our scoliosis is caused by postural misalignment and most often by a tight psoas. If your psoas is tight, it starts pulling on the lumbar curve in one direction. Sometimes people have a tight psoas on both sides, but very often they have one side that is tighter than the other. People often refer to their "shorter leg." From my perspective, that shorter leg is coming from a tight psoas. That tight psoas pulls the curve of the lumbar off center. This can create that scoliosis curve in the spine.

- **Tumors** can develop in the body that directly affect the spine and nerves creating all of the same symptoms commonly associated with sciatica and other lower back pain.

XII. SOLUTIONS FOR THE SPINE

We find that there is only one real way to make a spine happy. That is to retrain the way you walk and stand upright and learn how the spine works, developing the muscle tone to support it properly so that you can employ your newly developed patterns.

It always comes back to posture. Herniation, degeneration, stenosis, and spondylolisthesis – all of these can happen for many reasons but they often occur, or can be exacerbated, as a result of poor posture. The spine was designed to hold us up and bear and transfer weight down through the pelvis and the legs at the same time. It can't do this without all of the factors we have discussed; correct skeletal alignment and well-toned muscles prevent the breakdown of the body. Don't accept that everybody degenerates and loses their posture and becomes shorter. There is no reason for a bony degeneration to happen.

ALTERNATIVE THERAPIES

There are many avenues to pain relief and we strongly believe in the efficacy of certain alternative practices for bringing relief to spinal conditions. The key to this, and any approach to healing, is to become an active participant in your journey towards health. If you choose any of these methods, western or eastern, you have to become part of the solution.

Chinese Medicine- which includes Acupuncture, herbs, and bone-setting is as old as the hills and we think that any healing modality that has been around for three thousand years must have something going for it. As always, there is a caveat; these are not necessarily quick fixes, and will likely take many sessions and some time before they will be effective. Can they bring some immediate relief? Sure, but it is not meant as a short-term solution.

Network Chiropractic, a relatively new take on spinal analysis, can have excellent results when trying to realign the spine. This again is not a short- term solution. Depending on the severity of your injury and pain you may have to have a number of sessions a week until your spine finds its way to alignment. Once in alignment you can move to maintenance status and occasional treatments as determined by your practitioner.

Applied kiniesiology (AK)- one of our favorite approaches is the source of some controversy. It is a technique used to diagnose illness or choose treatment by testing muscles for strength and weakness. If you were to search AK online you will find an equal number of screeds claiming excellence and quackery. I have had a lot of personal experience with AK and think it is a great discipline.

Craniosacral Therapy is an alternative therapy used by many different body workers. Our parasympathetic nervous system, our system of relaxation, emanates from the cranium and the sacrum. A session involves the therapist placing their hands on the patient, tuning into the rhythm of cerebrospinal fluid as it runs through the brain and the spinal cord It is an extremely gentle and subtle practice that can ease the restrictions of nerve passages and help to realign the bones.

Our appreciation of eastern medicines doesn't mean we reject western medicine. In fact, I credit three necessary knee surgeries for starting me on my road to wellness. You might ask why it took three surgeries to figure out my problems, but you can just say I am a slow learner.

A PATIENT'S JOURNEY

Lets look at some of the medical options you might come across when you go to a doctor with issues of the spine.

Let's say that you go to see a doctor with a pain deep in your lower back that hasn't gone away for a long time and no diagnoses seems to fit. You've had x-rays that were negative, an MRI that shows nothing. You will most likely receive a referral for physical therapy that could prove very helpful but very often does not. Physical therapy is a great discipline but tends to treat the problem at its origin rather than treating the whole body. Which isn't to say it doesn't work but very often the relief provided is short term because the larger patterns that created the problem have not been dealt with.

Let's say physical therapy provided some relief but the pain and discomfort persists. At this point doctors often suggest an epidural injection similar to what a woman receives in labor. The shots often mix a steroid such as cortisone with an anesthetic like lidocaine. And sometimes they work. For different reasons, one of these shots can bring permanent relief. They almost always bring temporary relief which can often give the mind enough space to figure out a healing process, whether on your own or with a physical therapist, or other body worker. But very often these shots don't work and you will find yourself back in the doctors office filled with doubts

There are many doctors who will take the next step and suggest a morphine patch though we find that by the time you receive that suggestion you have been on the wrong train for too long and have to start looking for another route.

If your x-rays or MRI show some abnormality, then surgery becomes an available option. But this should always be the option of last resort. Back pain can take a long time to resolve itself but the fix won't last if you don't make changes to the patterns that allowed the problems to develop in the first place. That said, surgery, as a final option, can be a successful option.

There are numerous types of spinal surgeries. We'll lay out of few of them below.

Spinal Fusion is a technique where bone growth is stimulated to fill in the gap between two or more spinal segments to prevent motion that has been compressing the nerves. Metal is used to stabilize the spinal segments while bone eventually forms between the vertebrae. Spinal fusion has about an 80% success rate and is not always permanent. Depending on your age when you receive the procedure it might not last a lifetime

Dynamic Stabilization is an alternative to fusion surgery. This procedure attempts to provide stability to the spine without eliminating movement between the individual vertebrae

Lumbar Disc Replacement is another surgical option is to replace a disc entirely with a new one, which would allow movement at the level of replacement and not affect the spine above or below as function would remain exactly the same.

Spinal Discectomy is performed to remove a herniated disc from the spinal canal. When a herniation occurs, a fragment of the disc is dislodged. This fragment may press against the spinal cord or the nerves that surround the spinal cord. The treatment is to remove the fragment of disc that is causing the pressure on the nerve.

Laminectomy is a procedure to remove the portion of the vertebrae called the lamina. This becomes necessary if it is deemed that the lamina itself is pressing on the spinal cord. There are different types of laminectomy in which more or less of the bone is cut away.

Microdiscectomy removes a small portion of the bone over the nerve root providing more room for the nerve to heal. This procedure is more often that not used to alleviate sciatica, a shooting pain or numbness down the leg.

A NEW PARADIGM

In the next chapter we will provide a series of exercises designed to release tension filled spinal muscles, stretch tight spinal muscles and tone and strengthen weak muscle of the trunk that are necessary for proper support of the spine.

But first we will finish with a word to the wise. Wherever you end up on the spectrum of pain and healing there is a change that must take place.

We must become the architects of our own healing. Life is traumatic. From the big trauma of being born and taking our first breath to the lesser traumas of day-to-day life, we are here to be beaten up and to one degree or another develop an inner support system of healing. Like the pulsing of the heart and the ebb and flow of the tides, the body's trauma/healing interplay is as natural as breathing.

Our world has moved in strange directions in the last half-century. Every year Americans are turning more and more to surgical fixes for their injuries and ailments. With every ache and pain we take an advil or alleve. We are a society of external fixes, in search of a magic blue pill that will fix what ails us. The shift must be towards self-care and a belief that no one knows your body better than you. Doctors, nurses and body workers all serve a purpose. We need them to help facilitate our care and our health. But we have to take them off of the pedestal that we have created and become more pro-active in our own healing process.

What can and will fix us is easily found inside. We have a beautifully specific design that when embodied and enacted becomes a self-healing machine. Everyone knows what cancer is. Everyone knows what asthma is. Most people have heard of the word melanoma and can visualize a tumor but most people have not heard of the word psoas. Too many people don't know what the cervical spine bone is. We are painfully familiar with external circumstances or things that work upon us when we're really not all that familiar with the wonderful, magical body that we inhabit which can help us prevent so much of what ails us.

Our bones hold us up, our muscle move the bones after getting direction from the nerves. If the bones are aligned and the muscles toned, every movement you make will tone and stimulate all of your internal organs. Learn how your body works and discover that you are your best doctor. Cultivate a dialogue with your body that prioritizes instinct and trust. Get to know yourself. There is no better means to prevention. Be your own healer.

XIII. EXERCISES

There are any ways to exercise. In fact many people are exercising way more than they realize, if like me, you consider sitting at your desk exercise. It is an exercise that requires a counter stretch that is left forever wanting. But in the context of the series of exercises that we are presenting to you here, we will discuss touch on three types of physical work.

We love release work; the art of letting go. We present two release here for the back. Stretching once the body is released is very important but knowing when you are ready or how much stretch you want can be a science. And finally we offer some toning exercises. We are nothing without core tone. Bringing balance and tone to the musculature of the body is required for healthy living and graceful ageing.

A.   RELEASE

1. CONSTRUCTIVE REST POSITION (CRP)

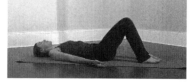

This is the main psoas release that we work with. It is a gravitational release of the psoas that allows the force of gravity to have its way with the contents of the trunk and the deep core.

- Lie on your back with your knees bent and your heels situated 12 to 16 inches away from your pelvis, in line with your sit bones.

- You can tie a belt around the middle of the thighs. This is a good thing to do, especially if you are weak in the inner thighs. You want to be able to really let go here and not have to think too much about the position of your legs.

- Then do nothing. You want to allow the body to let whatever happens to it come and go. Discomfort arises from conditioned muscular patterns. Try to allow the body to release rather than shift or move when unpleasant sensations arise.

- You are hoping to feel sensation that is something you can sit with and allow it to pass.

- Try to do this for 15 minutes a day, twice a day—in the morning and at night. If you have time, longer sessions are advisable.

But we are not here to suffer. If sensations come up and you feel that you just have to move, feel free to move, then come back to where you were and try again. It's possible that you'll do this exercise and not feel anything; that is fine also.

2. Cactus on the Back

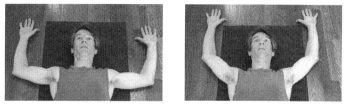

This falls somewhere between a release and a stretch and is not nearly as benign as some of these explorations. In fact, this can be very intense, though you won't be doing much.

- Lie flat on your back. If it is not comfortable to lie with the legs straight, roll up a blanket and place it under the knees. This will release the hamstrings and reduce the strain on the lower back.

- Bring your arms out to the side and bend your elbows to form a right angle with the arms.

- Lengthen the back of the neck and allow the spine to soften toward the floor. The lower back and neck should each have a gentle arch, but ideally the rest of the spine should have contact with the floor. Move very slowly.

- Once you get your spine into a good place, bring your awareness to the forearms, wrists and hands. Try to open the hands, extending the wrists and the fingers. Move very slowly.

- Once you get the arm to a good place return to the spine. Go back and forth between the two and allow the back of the body to lengthen, soften, and release.

B. STRETCH

1. Belt Stretch

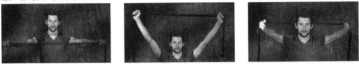

- This is a strong stretch of the Pectoralis minor at the front of the chest.

- Hold a belt or a broom stick with your hands wide apart. Bring the belt over your head and behind you keeping the arms straight. You may need to move your hands slightly further apart for them to stay straight.

- The key is for the head, neck and chest to remain still.

- Try to move both arms at the same pace.

- As this gets easier move the hands closer together.

2. QL on the back

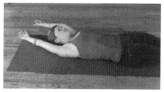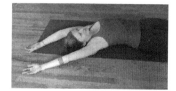

- Laying on your back extend your arms over your head.

- Stabilize your legs and pelvis and arc your trunk to the side

- You want to lengthen and stretch the area between the pelvis and the rib cage.

3. Side Stretch

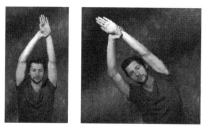

- Bring both hands over head. Stabilize the legs and pelvis. The pelvis should be pointing straight forward. Take hold of the right wrist in the left hand.

- Stretch to the left.

4. Car and Cow

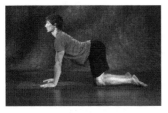 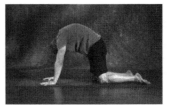

- Starting on you hands and knees begin to roll through the length of the spine from the tailbone at the base to the crown of the head at the top.

- Try to feel where you initiate the action from. Many times we start at the lower back. Try to tone your tail bone and move from the very base to the very top.

- If this is a comfortable shape try to figure out which parts of your spine work better than others. Feel, if you can, where you get stuck and what is fluid.

5. Sub Occipitals

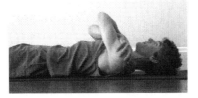

The sub occipital muscles connect the base of the skull to the top of the spine and are the only muscles in the body with an energetic connection to the eyes. They tend to be chronically short.

- Lie flat on your back and bring a small natural arch to your lower back. The legs should be straight; you can put a blanket under the knees if there is any strain on the lower back.

- Raise your arms to the sky, pulling your shoulder blades away from the floor. Try to let the upper spine settle onto the ground. Grasp each shoulder with the opposite hand.

- Lengthen the back of the neck as much as you can without closing off or creating discomfort at the front of the throat.

- Stay for three minutes to start, and try to build up to five minutes.

6. Cactus on the Belly

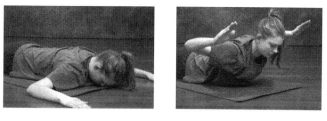

- Lie flat on your belly.

- Bring your arms out to the side and bend your elbows to form a right angle with the arms.

- Lengthen the back of the neck.

- Once you get your spine into a good place, bring your awareness to the forearms, wrists and hands. Everything is balance before you lift up, the forearms wrists and fingers are all balanced between extension and flexion.

- Lift the head neck and chest up off of the floor. Notice the difficulty in maintaining the balance in the different parts of the arm.

7. **Twist On Back**

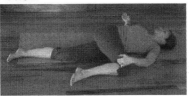

- Lay flat on your back.

- Draw the right knee into the chest and keep the left leg extending long on the floor. The left toes point straight up towards the ceiling.

- Begin to twist drawing the right knee across the left side of the body. The right knee can go over as much as possible, even reaching the floor if that work (or you could put a block or blanket or pillow under it).

- Let the left hand rest on the right thigh. Reach your right arm out to the right.

- Keep tone in the belly and look over the right shoulder. Slow down the breath and let the stretch happen.

- Change sides.

8. Back Stretch on the Belly

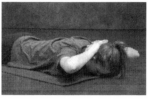 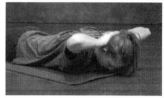

- Lie on your stomach. Interlace your fingers behind your head and lengthen the back of your neck up into your fingers.

- Draw the belly in and lift your trunk up off the floor, keeping your chin soft. The head neck and chest want to move in one piece.

- The elbows want to move up and out as you lift up. Let the hands rest on the head without pushing the head forward.

9. Winged Victory

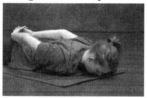 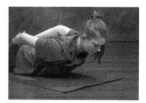

- Lie on your stomach. Interlace your fingers behind your back. Lengthen the back of your neck looking straight down.

- Draw the belly in and lift your trunk up off the floor, keeping your chin soft. The head, neck, and chest want to move in one piece.

C. STRENGTHEN

1. Pelvic Floor

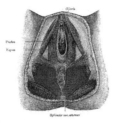

The pelvic floor is a large sling, or hammock, of muscles stretching from side to side across the floor of the pelvis. It is attached to your pubic bone in front, and to the coccyx (the tail end of the spine) in back. Make sure not to use your butt muscles in any of these exercises.

Doing these exercises correctly will help you find the correct placement of the pelvis which is key to all of the work we are trying to do.

When you tone or lift the pelvic floor the energetic quality should be a free lift up the central channel of the spine. If your pelvis is tucked under it is likely that your pubic bone will interrupt or stop the lift of the pelvic floor. Likewise, if your pelvis is rotated too far backwards you might feel that the sacrum or the back of the pelvis stops the upward flow of the pelvis floor. You know your pelvis is in the right place if the lift of the pelvic floor goes straight up the front of the spine.

There are three layers to the pelvic floor. You are trying to find the top layer, just slightly above holding in your pee (it can be very subtle)

- Tone your pelvic floor muscles, hold for a count of five. Do in sets of ten.

- Tone and lift your pelvic floor slowly, trying to stop and start as you go up, like an elevator stopping on several floors.

- If that seems easy enough try doing the opposite, lifting the pelvic floor, holding it at the top and lowering it incrementally.

- Practice quick contractions, drawing in the pelvic floor and holding for just one second before releasing the muscles. Do these in a steady manner aiming for a strong contraction each time building up to a count of fifty

2. Feet 3 Inches off the Floor

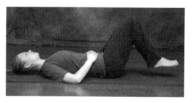

This exercise works the deep low belly muscle called the transverse abdominus. First, we're going to show how this muscle works and how another abdominal muscle, the rectus abdominus, works as well.

- Lie on your back on your mat. Bend your knees so that your feet are resting on the floor beneath your knees. Bring your hands onto the lower belly. Inhale and exhale. Inhale again and exhale but this time push the exhale at the end and see if you feel that your navel moves down to the spine and the muscle engagement is a feeling that wraps from the back to the front. Let that go.

- Now lift your head and shoulders and look at your knees. Here you should feel how when you lift the head and look at the knees, the belly pushes up into the fingers. Let the head release.

The first muscle that we engaged was called the transverse abdominis, a muscle that supports the lower back and wraps from the back to the front. The second muscle we engaged is called the rectus abdominis and connects the pelvis to the rib cage and moves in a direction straight up and down. We're going to try to isolate and engage only the deeper transverse muscle.

- Lift your right foot three inches off the floor and try to stabilize the spine as you lift the left foot three inches to meet it. Did the spine move up and the belly push up? Or did the spine actually stabilize and stay still? Release your feet.

- Starting with the second foot, lift the left foot three inches off the floor and lift the right foot three inches to meet it. Feel if the two sides were different.

- When lifting the feet without any movement in the belly or the spine becomes effortless and you can sustain it easily, bring the feet up to the height of the knees and parallel to the floor.

- When this becomes easy extend your knees forward two or three inches.

3. Block Between the Thighs on the Floor

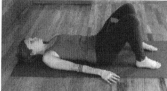 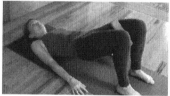

- Lay on your back with the knees bent and your feet flat on the floor.

- Place a block between your inner thighs. Engaging the inner thigh muscles against the block try to isolate them and use the quadriceps, and outer thighs, as little as possible.

- Don't grip your buttocks.

- Lift the hips up and continue to squeeze the block, drawing the low belly in to stabilize the spine.

- Hold for a count of 10 breaths. Try to hold longer as you feel stronger. Hold for less if you need to. See if you can build up staying for three minutes.

4. Core Twist (Internal and external Oblique)

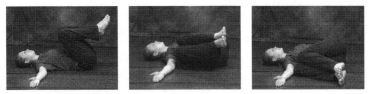

This is one of our mainstay poses used to work the abdominal muscles know as the internal and external obliques. There is a lot going on in this pose. The inner thighs should stay glued together and the shoulders are resisting the urge to pull off the floor as the legs go over to the opposite side.

- Lie down on your mat on your back. Bring your arms out to the side with the wrists at the height of the shoulders, like the letter T. Turn your palms up towards the ceiling.

- Draw your knees up into your chest.

- Attempting to move the knees up, bring your knees over towards the right inner elbow.

- Looking straight up the whole time, keep the legs together and slowly come back up to the center.

- In slow motion, move the knees to the left, again drawing them up towards the elbow.

- Coming back up to the center, keep squeezing the legs together and bring the knees up towards the nose.

- To go deeper in this exercise, you're going to come over to the right again and stop about two-thirds of the way down. Stop, hold, and squeeze the legs together and release the left side of the rib cage down towards the floor. Come back up to center slowly. Move to the left on an angle as slowly as you can, stop two-thirds of the way, hover and at the same time reach the right side of the rib cage down towards the floor.

- To go deeper still, the full pose is done with straight legs. The difficulty in this advanced version is keeping the legs straight, together, and moving up on an angle towards the finger tips. If the legs can't move on an angle towards the fingers you should only do this with the knees bent.

5. Boat

This classic yoga pose is another way to work the core and the advanced version brings the psoas in and out of engagement.

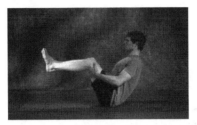

- Sit on the floor with your knees bent and the feet flat. Take hold of the back of your thighs and bring the feet up off the floor. That might be enough, or you might release the hands along side the knees.

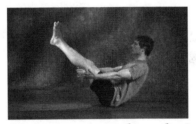

- If possible you can straighten the legs trying to bring the legs and trunk 60 degrees off of the floor. Keep the arms alongside the knees.

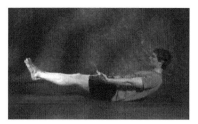

- As this gets easier, lean both the legs and the torso back to about 30 degrees. The back should round a bit and the work of the core should be stronger.

- Try to pull yourself back up to the original position. Repeat five times.

6. Knees One Inch off the Floor

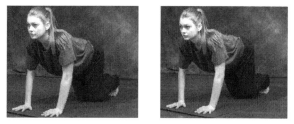

This exercise also works to stabilize the trunk. Engage your core and move the spine as little as possible when lifting the knees up.

- Start on your hands and knees.

- Soften your upper spine gently between the shoulder blades allowing them to soften onto the back.

- Tone the pelvic floor and low belly. Keeping the trunk stable lift your knees one inch off of the floor.

7. Forearm Plank

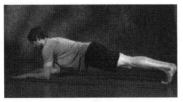

- Lie down on your belly with your elbows under your shoulders and your palms flat to the floor in front of you.

- Lift the hips up off of the floor bringing the ankles, hips, shoulders and ears into one straight line.

- If this is difficult begin by lifting the hips with the knees still on the floor and then try to lift the pelvis up.

- Be aware of the upper back. We have a tendency to round or push up the upper back and use the tightness of our chest muscles to hold us up. Try to broaden the upper chest and let the upper spine soften gently towards the floor.

8. Side Forearm Plank

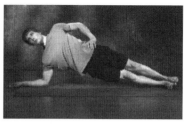

- Lie on your right side with your elbow under your shoulder and your hand lying at a right angle to your trunk with the palm flat to the floor.

- Bring your left hand to your left hip and flex your feet strongly.

- Try to lift your hips up off the floor trying to create a straight line from your right ankle to hip to shoulder. Do your best to keep your hips stacked on top of one another. The top hip tends to fall backwards.

- If this seems too hard, you can bring your left hand to the floor to try and help with the initial lift.

9. Bicycling the Legs

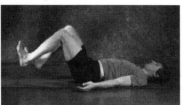

- Lay on your back and draw your right knee into your chest.

- Bring the left foot about a foot off of the floor.

- Begin to switch the position of the legs bring the left knee in and extending the right leg out.

- Try to keep the legs in line with the hips keeping them from extending out to the side.

- Be aware of your inner thighs and try to use them to help initiate the extension of the leg.

- If this is easy focus on moving the legs at the exact same time so that they cross in the exact middle. The dominant leg wants to move much faster.

10. Six Pack on a Block (Rectus Abdominus)

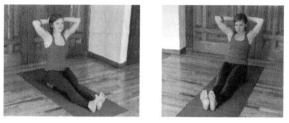

- Sit on a block with your legs outstretched and your fingers interlaced behind your head.

- Begin to lean backwards, shortening the distance between the rib cage and the pelvis engaging the muscle that runs up and down between them. The spine will round slightly into a crunch.

- Keep your heels on the floor. You can bend your knees slightly if the backs of your legs feel tight.

- Once this begins to get easier try to open the elbows wider while keeping the belly muscle engaged. This should bring your back muscles (lats) into play.

Acknowledgements

I have learned from so many people both in person and in print. Here is a short list of those who influenced this book.

Therese Bertherat, Bonnie Bainbridge Cohen, Irene Dowd, John Friend, Sandra Jamrog, , Genny Kapuler, Bessel van der Kolk, Liz Koch, Peter Levine, Tom Myers, Jenny Otto, Ida Rolf, Lulu Sweigard.

And to the many students who have been patient with me on my path to learning, you have been my true teachers and my true guides.

Thanks, as well, to our artists and models.

Artists: Frank Morris
             Mark Chamberlain

Models: Justine Cuelenaere
             CaitlinFitzGordon
             Ida FitzGordon
             Beth Hyde
             Jesse Kaminash
             David Martinez
             Christopher Moore
             Keith Yzquierdo.

32071750R00057

Made in the USA
Middletown, DE
21 May 2016